The Ketogenic Diet

30 Day Food Program
Easy and Fast
Avoid common mistakes
Lose weight and feel fit
Fast Weight Loss in 4 Weeks

Table of contents

Chapter 1

The ketogenic diet

The ketogenic diet allows the consumption of natural fats and proteins (meat, fish, poultry) and limited carbohydrates (sugars and starches). In a normal diet, carbohydrate consumption is very high (about 40-60% of calories), while the fat intake is limited. High carbohydrate diets have the effect of elevating blood sugar and insulin and over time, these levels increased to become chronic and cause the hunger effect as well as a series of pathological processes. In contrast, carbohydrate intake in a ketogenic diet is less than 4% of calories. When carbohydrate intake is low, meals are still delicious and filling. Hunger in this case goes away, and more importantly, this change of diet brings some beneficial effects on the metabolism of the human body, since it partially lowers the blood sugar level and consequently those of insulin. In this eBook, we will then talk about how the diet works, and we will provide the details for its correct implementation. The bottom line is that you can increase your energy and improve your health by simply changing the usual way of eating.

How the ketogenic diet works

As mentioned in the introduction, the limits of a diet with carbohydrates (sugar and starch), are important because when these foods are digested, they are divided into the body's blood (glucose). So, if you reduce your intake of carbohydrates by eating more fats and proteins, all this translates into a metabolic switch to as if it were a sort of primary fuel for burning fat. In this respect, a natural function is obtained since all the fat that is burned is converted into ketone bodies, and the blood glucose and insulin levels drop. The consequent increase in ketones brings benefits to the heart, muscles and brain. This state of "nutritional ketosis" is effective not only for proper nutrition but it is necessary to ward off various cancer pathologies.

Ketosis

At this point, those who read this eBook on the ketogenic diet will surely want to know what exactly ketosis is, and this is the basic phenomenon on which the diet is based, as can be seen from the denomination itself. The metabolic state of ketosis simply means that the amount of ketone bodies in the blood has reached higher than normal levels. When the body is in a ketogenic state, this means that the lipid energy metabolism is intact. The body will, therefore, begin to break down its body fat to feed the normal daily functions of the body itself. The question of the advantages of going into ketosis deserves an adequate answer, so it can be asserted that establishing this metabolic state of ketosis, even for a short period, gives significant benefits and excellent results to the subjects who have chosen it for lose weight. We can talk about 4 of the most significant advantages. The main one related to the state of ketosis is that it increases the body's ability to use fats as a fuel, which is generally mild in a carbohydrate-rich diet. When there is a high content of carbohydrates, the body can expect such a source of energy to enter the body. In the state of ketosis, the body must become efficient and instead use the fats to transform them into energy.

The second advantage dictated by the state of ketosis consists in the fact that it has a balancing effect on a protein level, starting from the assumption that adequate quantities of proteins and calories are being consumed equal to about 0.7 grams per kilo of body weight per day. Once in ketosis, the body prefers so-called ketones over harmful glucose. Since the body has abundant quantities of fat, this means that it is not necessary to oxidize proteins to generate glucose using a well-known process called gluconeogenesis. The third advantage is that basic ketosis keeps insulin levels low in the body, which causes greater lipolysis and free release of glycerol than a normal diet when insulin is around 80-120. Insulin has a blocking lipolysis effect, which can inhibit the use of fatty acids as energy. Furthermore, when insulin is brought to low levels, beneficial hormones are released into the body, such as growth hormones and other related factors. Finally speaking of the fourth advantage of the state of ketosis that is reached in a specific diet, we say that it consists in the fact that when entering the state of ketosis, ketones, in addition to high protein intake, also seem to suppress appetite, which instead it doesn't happen if the diet is rich in carbohydrates exactly the opposite happens, that is hunger increases out of all proportion.

The diet for diseases

Current research on cancer treatments considers the ketogenic diet, the results of which are extremely promising. The ketogenic diet for cancer therapy is a little different than the treatment for other diseases, the main idea behind the use of a ketogenic diet to treat cancer is that glucose cancer cells need to survive of healthy tissues. The big advantage of this treatment protocol is that it is not toxic to the body, but it is toxic to these cells, which means not allowing it to feed and therefore propagate. On the other hand, diabetics who are often advised to take more carbohydrates should be considered harmful to health because it leads to spikes in blood sugar, which in turn causes a greater need for drugs and insulin. A ketogenic diet reduces and, in many cases, eliminates the need to intervene with medicines, and reduces the number of units of insulin needed. For people with type 2 diabetes, the ketogenic diet reverses the

underlying insulin resistance which then causes the disease. However, it is important to know what this type of diet
is also suitable for people with type 1 diabetes as it can help reduce the number and severity of hypoglycemic episodes, reduce HbA1c values , and minimize future complications. When we talk about diet we think above all about how to lose weight without suffering from hunger, so the ketogenic diet seems the most suitable for this purpose; in fact, consuming few carbohydrates and fats has proven itself after careful studies, as the ideal solution for weight loss since the diet works with the biochemistry of the body instead of taking sides against it. Returning to the diseases that can be fought with a ketogenic diet, in that of Alzheimer's, ketones help to replenish the energy pathways of the brain and its health, and this translates into a better and functional memory.
Also, today the studies of the ketogenic diet have extended to other diseases with

awareness given the first results satisfactory that can be reversed or significantly improved by adopting such a diet. Finally, a word is worth spending on heart disease and neurology as the risk factors in the case of the former improve when the blood sugar and insulin levels drop through changes in the diet. For neurological disorders such as ALS, multiple sclerosis, and Parkinson's disease, research is showing that ketone bodies have a significant protective effect on the nervous system and slow the progression of these degenerative diseases of the nervous tissues.

Chapter 2

Planning the diet

A typical meal of the ketogenic diet includes about 90/150 grams of protein, and usually cooked in natural fats (for example, butter, lard, cream, olive oil, or coconut oil, with the addition of starch-free foods such as leafy vegetables such as lettuce, spinach, pumpkin, and cabbage,
so, if you are ready to get started, just check the diet plan, or draw up a list of low-carbohydrate foods. The ketogenic diet is therefore to improve well-being through a metabolic change in which the primary cellular fuel source passes from carbohydrate (glucose) fuels to fatty ones and their metabolism product called ketones. This result is obtained, in fact, through a process metabolic called ketogenesis, and with a relative state of the body called ketosis. Ketosis is simply a normal

metabolic path in which the body's cells use ketones to make energy instead of relying on sugar or carbohydrates. This consideration derives from the fact that humans have developed the evolutionary ability to burn ketones following an adaptation for periods when food was not available, such as after the period of, wars especially in Europe. Careful research has developed around ketosis since ketone bodies have revealed themselves in the human body. Increasing the rate of metabolic ketogenesis, therefore, serves to combat many diseases, because the presence of ketone bodies in the blood improves our health at the cellular level, in particular as a function of cellular energy pathways and mitochondrial health. The ketogenic diet is now used for the treatment of medical conditions such as diabetes, epilepsy, autism, Alzheimer's disease, cancer, and many others and much of the success of these treatments is rooted precisely in these cellular effects.

Advantages and disadvantages of the ketogenic diet

The dangers of low carbohydrate diets are few, but many people wonder if there are advantages or disadvantages to adopting them, especially for fears of getting fat and creating the ketosis process.

As for the former, most people have problems with a ketogenic diet plan because they are afraid of increasing the amount of fat they eat, especially saturated ones. The message that fat is bad is therefore present in the collective consciousness, but it is a lie since a high carbohydrate diet raises blood sugar and insulin levels leading the body to an inflammatory state. The standard diet offers, many foods high in sugar and rich in saturated fats, and in many studies, these two factors have been united, therefore, even if saturated fats lead to good health, the inflammation that causes diseases heartily they are due to their association with carbohydrates. A ketogenic diet plan which is high in saturated fat and very low in carbohydrates will, therefore, be able to reduce the aforementioned inflammation. Saturated fat is therefore not harmful in the context of a low carbohydrate diet. The ketogenic diet is therefore to be considered healthy because the intake of saturated fats increases HDL cholesterol, and, at the same time, a lower intake of carbohydrates decreases the levels of triglycerides. These two factors are the main suspects. It's proven that the cause of heart disease is precisely the consumption of high carbohydrates, instead of that of saturated fats. The best way before starting a diet is to get to know your body and do a complete blood test before starting a ketogenic diet program, fall at least 3 months, after which after this period the blood values must be checked again, even if you will notice the difference feeling much better after the first 30 days of the ketogenic diet. The latter must obviously be executed correctly; in fact, some people do not carry out the process of, ketosis especially if they do not consult a trusted doctor first, since, if the body is not perfectly healthy, there is a risk of running into kidney or heart problems. Although there is no evidence that many people do well by reducing their carbohydrate intake, I recommend it

is, however, that of not falling below 10-20 carbohydrates per day; in fact, it is clear that the ketogenic diet is very low in carbohydrates, but it is not a zero-carbohydrate diet. If you notice (after at least a month from the beginning of the diet) that you are not feeling well with very low carbohydrate levels, then it is sufficient to add others, such as eating sweet potatoes and other vegetables that tend to solve this small but important problem. They stay away from cereals and instead rely on vegetables, with a moderately high carbohydrate content (60-100 grams/day should, therefore, translate, in fact, health benefits.

General side effects

Switching to a ketogenic diet program can be uncomfortable at first, as the body's metabolism is reluctant to burn fat instead of using glucose instead, which means that there may be some common side effects by applying the ketogenic diet. In this regard, here is a list of those that could already manifest themselves from the first week or so. During this time cut carbohydrate intake, blood sugar levels can cause mild insulin overload and reactive hypoglycemia. This usually happens to people who are severely insulin resistant. It, therefore, takes about 2-3 days to burn all the stored glycogen (in the muscles and in the liver), and the main anytime, the symptoms are dizziness, tremors, the classic heart in the throat, and more. As mentioned above, the dangers of low carbohydrate diets are based on false beliefs and unfounded fears, generally communicated by people who have a limited understanding of how important it is instead to keep their values leveled down, and in this consideration are not helped by the advertisements of well-known brands of food products that are trying their best to enter the market and create misleading and untruthful advertisements asserting that the foods on offer are healthy.

At this point, let's go back to our ketogenic diet plan by saying first that there are many ways to implement it so that aside from keeping carbohydrates low with higher fat levels, the plan for a ketogenic diet requires monitoring the amounts of carbohydrates in the foods consumed and reducing their carbohydrate intake to about 20-60 grams per day. For some people, less than 100 grams per day may work, nevertheless less carbohydrate intake is too high to achieve the ketosis necessary for it to function properly. In addition, also insulin requirement should be guided by a specific target such as weight ideal body or lean body mass. However, protein intake also depends on height, gender, and the number of daily gymnastic exercises. Eating too much protein, interfere with the ketosis process, which therefore must be well supported by a healthy and unhealthy physique.

Chapter 3

Menu of the ketogenic diet

In this chapter, we deal with drawing up an example of a menu suitable for a ketogenic diet by proposing the three-day one which in summary manages to explain the concept of the functionality of the diet itself and the necessary supply of foods capable of promoting ketosis.

Day 1

The grams of protein, in this case, is a bit higher but the intake of calories and the percentage of protein is perfect when compared with the percentage of fat. Thus, a breakfast of scrambled eggs with the addition of cream and onions, and 3 slices of bacon are ideal. For lunch instead of the chicken breast seasoned with a green salad, a drizzle of vinegar oil, and a little celery year well. In the evening for dinner, a cream of mushroom mixed with broccoli serves to keep the calorie intake started early in the morning constant.

Day 2

On the second day for breakfast, 120 grams of minced meat mixed with some spices, a little chopped onion, are then created and fried meatballs are created in butter or olive oil. As a drink, the advice is to consume an unsweetened herbal tea or coffee with cream. For lunch 120 grams of baked fish seasoned with butter sauce and a bowl of cauliflower, chopped and salted in butter or olive oil. As a side dish of green salad, it is more than enough species if accompanied by fresh cheese, mind like drinks water, or other as long as without sugar they are fine. For dinner, about 180 grams of pork shoulder, always chopped with cabbage sautéed in butter or olive oil, are perfect for ending the day.

Day 3

On the third day for breakfast are indicated sausages (max 100 gr), a soft-boiled egg, two slices of cheese and whipped cream and as a drink of unsweetened tea or correct coffee with cream. For lunch, on the other hand, 120 grams of smoked turkey, a cup of pumpkin sautéed in butter or olive oil, a vegetable salad low in carbohydrates, and with a high-fat dressing and as a drink, natural or carbonated water are ideal. Finally, for dinner 120 grams of salmon, cream of parmesan sauce, 2 cups of spinach sautéed with onions and garlic, Roman lettuce with low carbohydrate content, and with a high-fat dressing. Water, coffee, or tea are the recommended drinks to accompany the meal. These listed so far are just a few examples of what the menu of a ketogenic diet is. However, as already mentioned above, it is important to consume proteins, adding fat (within a certain calorie limit), and also the choice of vegetables containing a low carbohydrate content is ideal to complete the meal.

Chapter 4

Fats, vegetables and drink

Fats and oils

Since most of the calories in a ketogenic diet come from dietary fats, the choices must be made in the right way, and since many people cannot tolerate a large amount of vegetable oil, mayonnaise, or olive oil, this is a good one. what, since vegetable oils are rich in polyunsaturated Omega-6 fatty acids found in walnut, margarine, soybean oil, sunflower oil, safflower oil, corn oil, and canola oil or all ready to generate inflammation in the body. However, there are some essential polyunsaturated fats and these are Omega 6 and Omega 3. The intake of both types must however be balanced, and therefore only about one teaspoon a day is needed. Eating salmon, tuna and shellfish will provide an excellent balance of Omega 3 fatty acids, for example, and are an important part of a list of low carbohydrate foods. Some walnuts or mayonnaise will also provide Omega 6. If you don't like fish, then only consider small quantities for an essential Omega 3 fat supplement. Saturated and monounsaturated fats, such as butter, macadamia nuts coconut, avocado, and egg yolks are more easily tolerated by most people, and since they are chemically stable, they are less inflammatory. Fats and oils can also be combined with sauces, seasonings, and added to other meals. Keeping cold-pressed oils such as almonds and flax seeds in the refrigerator also helps to avoid rancidity. Vegetable heating oils are to be avoided; therefore, it is advisable to use clean and non-hydrogenated lard, coconut oil, and olive oil for frying since they have very high smoke points. As regards meat, both veal and game are good, while for fish, seafood of all kinds is preferred, anchovies, cod, halibut, squid, herring, mackerel, salmon, sardines, snappers, trout, and tuna, the latter like salmon are also good canned. To avoid are fried fish whether they are clams, crabs, lobsters, scallops, shrimps, squid, mussels, and oysters. As for whole eggs, they can be prepared in many ways such as deviled, fried, boiled, to make omelets, poached, scrambled, or soft-boiled.

Fresh vegetables

Most vegetables that are not starchy are also low in carbohydrates and ideal are organic vegetables to avoid dangerous pesticide residues. Therefore, avoiding vegetables that are rich in starch is important and among these, we find corn, peas, potatoes, and most of the squash as they are also very high in carbohydrates. The same applies to some types of sweet vegetables and vegetables such as tomatoes, carrots, pepper, and summer pumpkins. This list is not complete, so if there is a green vegetable that you like and that is low in carbohydrates, then it will be welcome for your ketogenic diet. Among the other recommended types, it is worth listing them starting with alfalfa sprouts, all green leafy vegetables, asparagus, beets, Brussels sprouts, celery, cucumbers, dandelions, garlic.

chicory, endive, escarole, fennel, radicchio, mushrooms, olives, radishes, and turnips.

Walnuts and seeds are instead excellent impregnated ideal for seasoning roasts and are also very rich in calories even if, to tell the truth, they also have a higher content of carbohydrates per serving. Macadamia, pecans, and almonds are the ones that have the lowest net carbohydrate content and therefore they can be eaten in small quantities, further reducing the intake of other types such as cashews, pistachios, and chestnuts which are richer in carbohydrates.

Drinks

The drinks to be consumed before, during and after meals are manifold; in fact, we find decaffeinated coffee, decaffeinated tea (unsweetened), a herbal tea (unsweetened), water, carbonated or flavored water (bitter), lemon and lime juice provided in small quantities, almond milk, coconut and soybeans, ns as long as they are not sweetened. Finally, as far as sugars are concerned, there are alternative sweeteners and among these, we find those based on dextrin malts, such as stevia, erythritol, xylitol, and fructose.

Chapter 5

Thirty-day menu

Week 1

Simplicity is the key for those just starting on a low carbohydrate diet; in fact, it is not a relationship between the kitchen and an essay, since getting rid of the desire to eat some foods will not be difficult since the 30-day program provides abundant and satisfying meals for the palate, not to mention that even smoothies can be deliciously prepared with fruit and vegetables, ideal for any time of day, especially when the desire to add something pending a new meal takes over and leftovers will also be another thing to be taken into consideration. All this is not only easier for those who practice the ketogenic diet, but also because it avoids the hassle of cooking the same food more than once. For example, breakfast is something that you can do every day with leftovers, and where you don't have to worry every morning about making it artificially, so just take some food out of the fridge and you're done! When starting a ketogenic diet, the first signs of ketosis are known as "keto flu" in which headaches, clouding of the brain, fatigue, and other mild and annoying similar manifestations can irritate your body. Making sure to drink plenty of water and eat plenty of salt is the first important step. The ketogenic diet is based, in fact, also on a diuretic process that goes beyond normal, so it must be taken into consideration that maintaining your body with a good intake of salt and the intake of high enough water is very important, as it allows the body itself to rehydrate and recover the electrolytes expelled during extraordinary urination. Doing so will help fight the aforementioned headache and other annoyances, if not get rid of them completely, and if necessary, it is advisable to drink water with a sprinkling of salt. In this case, just keep drinking water (at least 4 liters per day), and continue to eat salt. However, if you are concerned about the high blood pressure caused by salt, it is important to know that recent reports have shown that sodium intake and blood pressure are not as correlated as previously believed.

For breakfast, if you want to prepare something fast, easy, tasty, and natural, the suggestion is to start the first day from a weekend. In this way, it is possible to prepare on the weekend and with more time available, given the absence of work commitments, something that will last for the whole week which is the first is all based on simplicity. Even for lunch y, you can use simple things; most of the time, it will be necessary to prepare salad and meat, although, for the l, latter, it is important to know that you can also use leftover meat or easily use that canned can and the same for fish. If you use canned meat, however, it is advisable to read the labels to get information on what you consume and above all to avoid those that have additives often used as preservatives that harm your health regardless of the type of diet chosen. Dinner will instead be a combination of green leafy vegetables (normally broccoli and spinach), with a little meat, and also, in this case, we will go on high fat and protein in moderation.

Week 2

Since the first week is over, you can start with the second week and in this case, we can keep it simple again for breakfast by introducing coffee but not absolute; in fact, it is a mixture based on coconut oil, butter, and cream to be added precisely in coffee.

This concoction is not as strange as it seems, since butter, after all, is made of cream. So, when they blend oil and butter and cream, together they add a nice taste to the coffee.

For breakfast, we are therefore going to change a bit, and if you are not a coffee lover, you can try the same way with tea.

Even in the second week, as regards lunch, you can keep it simple; in fact, you can have more meat than the previous day with the only preparation of green vegetables and high-fat seasonings (or pinzimonio) which are fundamental for the success of a ketogenic diet. In this way, you can balance the fats with the amount of protein which is very important. For dinner, once again, it will be quite simple: meats, vegetables, high seasonings based on fats are the masters, even if as has been noted also for this second week of the diet, no dessert appears after the meals, but we invite you to read with confidence this eBook dedicated to the thirty-day menu since the first nice surprises in this regard come from the third week.

Week 3

This week we use light and fast meals and specifically, it is about getting a full fat in the morning and that must last until dinner time. From this point of view, not only are there a myriad of health benefits, but it is also easier to choose the eating program (and the cooking methods); in fact, the suggestion is to make (rather, drink) breakfast at 7 in the morning and then eat dinner at 7 in the evening. Keeping 12 hours between meals will help put the body in a state of fasting in which it can break down the extra fat that is stored to get the energy it needs instead. When you are in ketosis, the body in itself already imitates a state of fasting and without any blood glucose, and in this way, fats are used to develop energy necessary for the body. Having said that, one might think that it is a great and ingenious found to lose weight quickly, it is also true, however, that one must take into account that later, it is necessary to eat extra fat to keep the hunger mode under control. This sort of intermittent fasting brings several benefits and some include lipid blood levels, longevity, and much needed mental clarity, in everyday life, at work and why not to tackle the diet with the right spirit. However, if it turns out that you can't have a quick meal, it's not a big deal; in fact, just go back to the first week and experience meals as you see fit. The ketogenic diet with the thirty-day plan can, therefore, be defined as the one that allows you to eat everything but in small portions or at least divided by time slots, which does not involve stress and the results are seen, and without worrying about cooking more appetizing dishes, since they already are. After having dutifully lingered for a long time in the third week which in our opinion represents the fulcrum of the ketogenic diet, however, let's see in detail what to eat for breakfast and dinner. So, starting with full fat, like breakfast, this time there will be twice the amount of correct coffee (or tea) which means doubling the amount of coconut oil, butter, and cream, and maybe even adding something caloric, such as a bar of dark chocolate usually bitter compared to milk chocolate, so that you can arrive at dinner without problems. Remember that water remains an indispensable element to better hydrate the body to compensate for some hunger symptoms after a couple of hours, and at the same time purify it. Meats, vegetables, and fats are allowed at dinner, but the real surprise comes from the desserts; in fact, this week you can create low carbohydrate content by eating great delicacies, which will refresh your stomach, and above all your mind.

Week 4

This week we are getting ready to be a little tighter with fasting. After the intermittent week, now we must skip breakfast and lunch. In this case, water is the best ally! We must not forget that you can drink coffee, tea, flavored water, and the like to obtain precious and liquid nutrients. This undoubtedly represents a big problem, but you have to get used to it and if you succeed, your efforts will reward you. In the evening, dinner with a fairly substantial and protein-rich dessert such as chicken, abundant, and with a load of vegetables.

The ideal recipes for the ketogenic diet

In this eBook, we could not fail to recommend some suitable recipes to optimize the ketogenic diet, so in this sequence, we list some very suitable and particularly tasty.

Cabbage and poached eggs

Poached eggs are perfect but are usually served with a carbohydrate such as a salty muffin. Well, this recipe replaces the unsuitable carbohydrate for the ketogenic diet with organic cabbage to obtain for example a breakfast that we can call a superfood. Preparation is not difficult so just follow the guidelines below.

To begin with, melt a spoonful of butter in a small pan and then add a peeled clove of garlic, leaving to cook for about a minute. At this point add about 60 grams of raw cabbage, washed and cut, after which the whole is covered with a lid and cooked for about 5 minutes, stirring occasionally. While this cooking is taking place, it is necessary to separate an egg into two bowls, and where there is only the white one must add another spoonful of butter and then fry the other egg as well. For the accompanying sauce, just melt 2 tablespoons of butter with 1 tablespoon of coconut cream, using a small food processor, and adding the rest of the remaining egg yolk, a pinch of salt, and a good grated pepper fresh black, until it forms a homogeneous cream.

To serve, just cover the plate with the cooked cabbage, add the fried egg on top, and then add a lot of hollandaise sauce, so it's called the one we just created.

Chia seed pudding

Chia seeds are very rich in proteins, ideal for a hearty breakfast and to keep the heart-healthy, especially for the high content of omega-3 as well as many fibers, which fill the stomach until lunchtime. Also, it is incredibly versatile from a culinary point of view. The preparation is as follows: First, you need, ed to combine about 30 grams of chia seeds with 1 cup of coconut milk and ½ tablespoon of your favorite sweetener. Then leave the mixture to rest in the refrigerator for at least one night and wake up in the morning eating a delicious chia pudding. Depending on the choice of milk and sweeteners (excellent honey, but maple syrup also works well), this breakfast offers infinite variations; in fact, do you want to add almonds or coconut flakes for example? You can do it without any problem!

Muffins with vegetables and cheese

A low carbohydrate breakfast is super easy to prepare and consists of using vegetables, eggs, cheese and muffins. In this regard, the recipe echoes: Sprinkle a muffin pan with a little cooking oil, after which you have to scramble the eggs with milk, cheese, and vegetables, and then just pour a little of the mixture obtained in the muffin mold and cook it in the oven at 200 degrees for about 20 minutes.

Superfood soup

A soup, ideal to eat at lunchtime, is one of the best ways to take a break from stress. It is enough to fill a nice hot bowl with typical products of vegetarian cuisine. In detail, the preparation takes place as follows; Peel and finely dice a medium white onion and 2 cloves of garlic and place them both in a pan with about 30 grams of butter or with coconut oil. At this point, you have to cook it on medium-high heat until they are a little golden brown. In the meantime, at least 150 grams of watercress and 200 of fresh or frozen spinach must be washed and set aside. Then cut a medium head of cauliflower into small florets and place it in the pan with the browned onion. At this point, add a crumbled bay leaf and cook for about 5 minutes, stirring often. When cooked, pour

spinach and watercress and cook until wilted or for about 2-3 minutes. Once this operation is done, pour a liter of vegetable broth and bring it to the boil, making the cauliflower cook inside until it becomes soft enough. The next step involves the addition of a cup of coconut milk, s, salt and pepper, after which it is removed from the heat and blended until it is creamy. The dish is then eaten cold, and it is also important to know that the recipe, although elaborated, is valid and advantageous, since it can also be kept for up to 5 days in the fridge.

Finally, after listing the recipes for breakfast and lunch of a ketogenic diet, we conclude this quick overview, with two other dishes to eat for dinner and precisely one based on meat and the other of fish.

Steak with mushrooms

To prepare this succulent dish to be eaten for dinner in the ketogenic diet program, you must first preheat the oven to about 250 degrees, then with your hands sprinkle both sides of the steak with salt and pepper. At this point, put it in a pan

a tablespoon of butter until it boils, then cook the steak for at least two minutes on each side and then immediately put it in the oven until it becomes crispy. Once this is done, we put them aside for a moment and pour some white wine into the pan to recover the leftovers of the meat and the seasoning in which we cooked it, until it evaporates. At this point in the same pan add the previously boiled mushrooms and everything must be poured on the steaks which in this way are beautiful and ready to be consumed and to delight the palate.

Baked salmon

Salmon is another ideal food to prepare a dinner suitable for the ketogenic diet, especially for the high amount of omega 3 fats. One of the easiest ways to prepare is to take a glass dish and marinate the salmon with 2 finely chopped cloves of garlic, 6 tablespoons of extra virgin olive oil, dried basil, salt (at least a teaspoon), black pepper, the juice of about two lemons and finely chopped fresh parsley. The salmon fillets are then left in this state for about a couple of hours, after which they must be laid on aluminum foil and browned in the oven previously kneaded at 180 degrees and cooked for at least 40 minutes.

In the margins of this eBook, we just have to list some excellent smoothies that may become indispensable during the aforementioned thirty-day period and precisely in the fourth week, where, as seen, both breakfast and lunch must be skipped and were at the same time, it was recommended to drink a lot. Starting from the latter, here is a list of 4 excellent smoothies ideal for the ketogenic diet.

The ideal smoothies for the ketogenic diet

When the months when the greatest quantities of fresh fruit are available, it is important to know that the latter can be used not only to prepare fruit salads but also to create very tasty and above all healthy smoothies, as they are rich in vitamins and many antioxidants, essential to make the body feel good. The smoothies are ideal for all diets and in particular for the ketogenic one since they can be inserted in the intervals between a meal and the other species when the 30-day diet program as already mentioned in the previous chapters of this eBook, gets harder to be implemented and this is evident in particular in the fourth week whereas we have seen you can only have dinner, and therefore a smoothie instead of breakfast and lunch do not create performance problems nor does it cause damage to health or cause overweight since it's made with moisturizing liquids and with natural sugars such as fructose. So, if you have excellent fresh and perhaps organic fruit, you can certainly not waste anything, not even the peel of apples, pears, peaches, apricots, plums and many others. Preparing smoothies can at the same time become not only a good daily habit but also a way to distract yourself from the stress of the diet that you are practicing, and with the possibility of personalizing it as best at that moment your mind and above all the palate they desire.

Banana smoothie

To prepare this delicious milkshake which, among other things, in the summer also helps to combat the typical exhaustion of the season and prevents adductor night cramps because rich in potassium, it is only complicated; in fact, just add a banana appropriately cut into small slices in a glass with inside the natural orange juice, the pulp of an avocado and a light sprinkling of powdered ginger. Everything is then placed in a blender or in a d p by operating them for a few minutes just the time necessary to obtain the creaminess and consistency that is best desired. Depending on your personal ta can also add more to the banana-based smoothie such as, for example, the juice of half a lemon, and a few meta leaves just to make it fresher.

Smoothie with blackberries and raspberries

After taking a healthy walk on a mountain path and with an appetite for a thousand, which we cannot dampen because we are forced to follow the predetermined ketogenic diet, there is nothing better than preparing a blackberry and raspberry smoothie. Specifically, it is a matter of collecting as you approach home, these juicy, delicious and precious berries that are also rich in antioxidants, and which we can then blend by simply adding water and at most, a half teaspoon of brown sugar taking into account that white sugar is absolutely not recommended the ketogenic diet. However, it should be emphasized that these typical berries are already sufficiently sweetened, so the addition of other sweeteners could prove superfluous.

Fruit, vegetable and vegetable smoothie

Also, many vegetables and vegetables, in addition to the aforementioned fresh fruit, are ideal for preparing tasty smoothies to be used during long waiting periods between meals, imposed by the ketogenic diet. Green leafy vegetables and some vegetables such as carrots (suitably boiled and then cooled) are suitable for a smoothie rich in vitamins. According to your personal tastes, even cabbage leaves, the same carrots, a few slices of banana, Greek or soy yogurt and freshly pressed orange juice, can be placed in the blender, all enough to create a drink consistent and very welcome especially on very hot summer days. It is above all ideal for combating dysentery, another typical seasonal phenomenon often dictated by the consumption of non-fresh food or by the intake of cold drinks.

Avocado and basil smoothie

Whisk the pulp of a fairly ripe avocado and at least five or six fresh basil leaves together with a glass of soy milk or rice, a teaspoon of lemon juice and one of brown cane sugar. You get a truly refreshing drink, as well as a vitamin, perhaps, with the addition of a couple of ice cubes, ideal to be consumed on hot summer days.

Coffee smoothie

As we have seen in the previous chapters and especially in the thirty-day menu, coffee is one of the drinks that is recommended for all breakfasts, so it is also worth listing it as a basic product to create a tasty and refreshing liquid for hot and muggy days summer and not only; in fact, even at breakfast you can opt for this type of smoothie, making it in various ways and drawing on the products that the ketogenic diet such as coffee itself allows you to use. An example is to take half a Moka-pot of coffee just out of the mocha, put it in the blender, and add a half glass of Greek yogurt and bitter cocoa. All suitably blended, especially with ice cubes, becomes creamy and shaken-like, that is, with a velvety appearance and a unique taste, such as to lick even what remains inside the small rotating blades of the blender. An alternative is to add only fresh eggs of the day to the coffee (possibly bio-type to avoid risks of salmonella) and prepare substantial and tasty eggnog, or a healthy drink, typical of farms. As well as widespread at the time of our grandparents.

Green tea smoothie

The bland smoothies mainly based on grass and water, as for coffee, are among the most suitable as a drink to be consumed during a ketogenic diet, especially as we have seen previously in the absence of solid meals. What involves the use of green tea is simple, but the beneficial properties of this plant are remarkable, so much so that it always finds its rightful place in all the various types of diets. Green tea, to name just a few of its beneficial properties, is above all an excellent antibacterial; in fact, its beneficial action is particularly reflected in the mouth and teeth. The substances contained in it are, in fact, able to counteract the bacteria of the oral cavity, as well as being ideal for preventing the formation of caries. Green tea is above all a high concentrate of antioxidants, such as polyphenols and bioflavonoids. These two antioxidants, like many others, are indispensable in the human organism to slow down the aging of cells, favor tissue regeneration and at the same time effectively counteract free radicals, which in turn are responsible for the main degenerative diseases such as multiple sclerosis and Parkinson's disease. Finally, green tea is highly valued by nutritionists because it is considered an excellent ally against obesity thanks to its beneficial properties. The experts at Penn State University have identified in this herb substances capable of burning excess fat in the human body, and of reducing the adipose state of the tissues. If one plus one equals two, then it seems right to us in the ketogenic diet, do not exclude a green tea-based smoothie, perhaps with the addition of a healthy spoonful of bee honey, or simply as an aggregating liquid for all the other types of smoothies, whether based on fruit or vegetables.